better nutrition *magazine* presents

RELAX

by **SHERRY TORKOS, BSc Phm**

better nutrition healthy living guide

Published by:
Active Interest Media, Inc.
300 N. Continental Blvd., Suite 650
El Segundo, CA 90245

This booklet is part of the *Better Nutrition Healthy Living Guide* series. For more information, visit www.betternutrition.com. Better Nutrition magazine is available at fine natural health stores throughout the United States. Design by Aline Design: Bellingham, Wash.

RELAX

CONTENTS

better nutrition healthy living guide

Introduction
Stressful Living

In our fast-paced society with our busy lifestyles, increasing work demands, and social and economic challenges, it is not surprising that stress has become a burgeoning force in our lives. Stress is something that each and every one of us has to deal with every day. How we manage our stress is critical. Without the proper coping mechanisms and lifestyle approaches, stress can take a serious toll on our health.

As a pharmacist, I often hear people say, "I'm stressed out." Stress leads to numerous health problems, which send people to the doctor's office and ultimately to the pharmacy for one of the many available prescription tranquilizers, sedatives, or antidepressant medications. However, I feel prescription drugs should be a last resort. There are so many other, safer ways to manage stress.

There are countless books on the subject of stress management, and while some are helpful, others can be overwhelming and require drastic lifestyle changes that in themselves can be stressful. In this booklet, I will share with you my practical and proven methods for managing stress through dietary strategies, exercise, relaxation techniques, and nutritional supplements. As stress is an inevitable part of our lives, effective coping strategies are essential for maintaining physical and emotional well-being. Fortunately, adopting these strategies is not going to be as difficult as you may think.

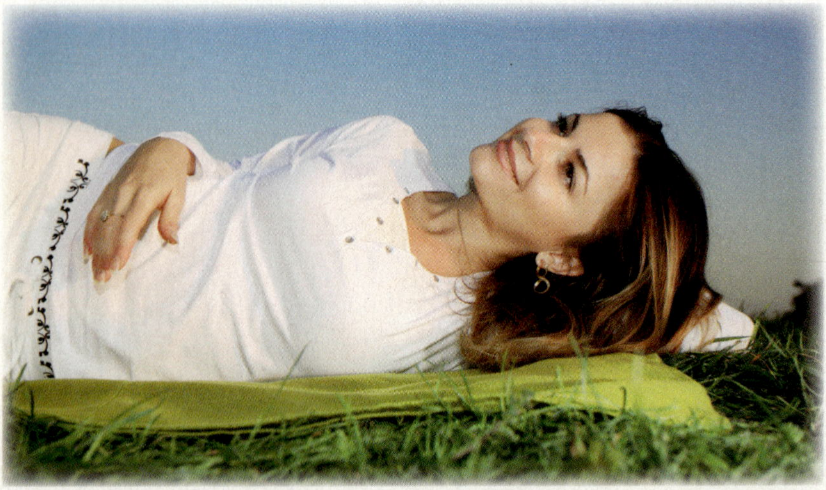

Chapter One
Understanding Stress

We often throw around the term "stress" in reference to unpleasant experiences, situations, or people, but what exactly is the definition of stress? The first person to coin the term "stress" was Hans Selye, MD, PhD, a Canadian endocrinologist. In 1936 he defined stress as "the non-specific response of the body to any demand for change." In laboratory experiments, Selye discovered that animals subjected to physical and emotional stimuli such as blaring light, loud noise, or extreme temperatures all exhibited the same effects — namely, stomach ulcerations, shrinkage of the thymus gland, and enlargement of the adrenal glands. In further experiments, he demonstrated that persistent stress could cause animals to develop diseases similar to those seen in humans, such as heart attacks, stroke, kidney disease, and rheumatoid arthritis. Selye's theories attracted worldwide attention, and stress soon became a popular buzzword.

Bad Stress, Good Stress

Since people viewed stress as some unpleasant threat, Selye subsequently had to create a new word, "stressor," to distinguish stimulus from response. Stress was the body's reaction to a situation or event, which is the stimulus (the stressor). Stress was generally considered as being synonymous with distress, or as a physical, mental, or emotional strain or tension. Thus, stress was put in a negative light, and its positive effects ignored. Stress can be a good thing, such as when it motivates people to accomplish more.

The Stress Response

The hypothalamic-pituitary-adrenal axis (HPA axis) system is how the body responds to stress. Selye first described this system while identifying the three stages of the stress response: alarm, resistance, and exhaustion.

When the threat or stressor is identified or realized, the body responds in a state of alarm. Stress hormones called catecholamines (adrenaline and noradrenaline) and glucocorticoids (cortisol) are released. These hormones, which are secreted by the adrenal glands, function to prepare the body to fight, and hence this response is known as the fight-or-flight response. When this occurs, our body enters a catabolic state, where our fuels (glucose, fats, and amino acids) are broken down to provide energy. Heart rate, blood pressure, blood volume, and pulmonary (lung) tone increase to enhance the function of the heart and lungs. Muscle tone increases to improve strength and performance.

The second stage is known as resistance. If the stressor persists, it becomes necessary to attempt some means of coping with the stress. Although the body begins to try to adapt to the strains or demands of the environment, the body cannot keep this up indefinitely, so its resources are gradually depleted.

The third and final stage is exhaustion. The body's resources are depleted and the body is unable to maintain normal function. At this point, the initial stress symptoms, such as sweating and increased heart rate, may reappear.

This stress response, an innate mechanism, was designed to help us cope with short bursts of stress, such as running away from a predator. We often hear that cortisol is a bad thing, but in reality we could not survive without cortisol, or the other stress hormones. The problem is that our bodies have not adapted to handle a continuous onslaught of stress (and continuous release of stress hormones). As a result, this reaction wreaks havoc on almost every system in our bodies. When stress is chronic, it results in damage to vital glands, including the adrenal and thymus glands. The immune system becomes exhausted and its function is impaired. The obvious effects of chronic stress are mental impairment, increased risk of illness and infections, ulcers, and heart and digestive problems. Many aspects of health become compromised as a result of chronic stress.

Are You Stressed?

Some of us seem to handle stress better than others. A lot of that has to do with our personality type, our coping skills, and how we are conditioned from a young age to deal with stressful life situations.

We all know people who seem to be stressed out. The overachiever, the "type A" personality, the perfectionist, the person who easily panics: these people always seem to be wound up and ready to explode. But there are also people who, on the outside, seem to handle stress well, but inside they worry and suffer effects of stress such as anxiety and sleeplessness.

According to a 2007 survey by the American Psychological Association, nearly one-third of U.S. adults report "extreme stress." Also in this survey, it was revealed that:

- Nearly one in five (17 percent) respondents reach their highest stress level 15 or more days per month.
- Almost half (48 percent) reported that their stress level has risen over the last five years.

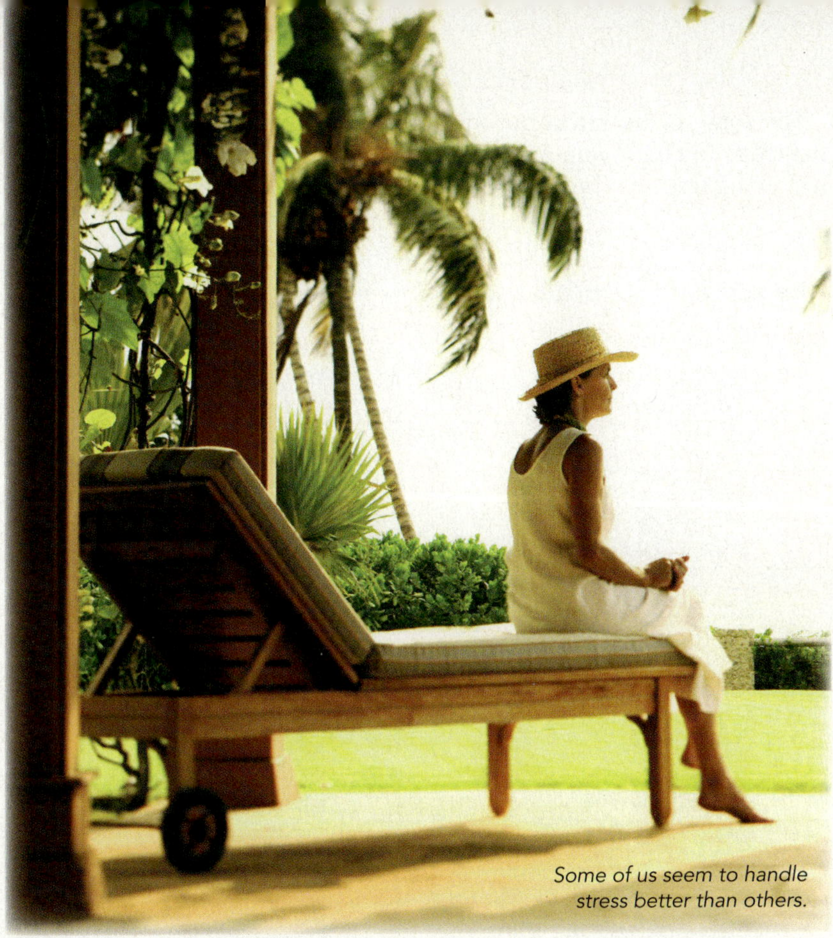

Some of us seem to handle stress better than others.

- More than three out of four participants (77 percent) said that within the previous month, they had experienced physical problems due to stress. Those problems included fatigue, headache, upset stomach, muscle tension, change in appetite, teeth grinding, change in sex drive, and feeling dizzy.
- Stress kept nearly half of participants awake at night during the previous month. They reported losing 21 hours of sleep during that month.
- Almost half of participants (43 percent) said they had overeaten or eaten unhealthy foods because of stress in the previous month. Candy and chocolate were the most popular comfort foods.

As for the underlying causes of stress, almost three-quarters of participants noted work stress and money stress as the most significant stressors. Workload, children, health concerns, and housing costs stressed about half of the participants.

For some of us, stress becomes a chronic problem that goes unrecognized. To check your stress level, take a few minutes to complete the following test.

What's your stress index?

(Mark each box that applies and then total the number of boxes marked.)

Do you frequently:

	Neglect your diet?		Have few supportive relationships?
	Try to do everything yourself?		Get too little rest?
	Blow up easily?		Ignore stress symptoms?
	Seek unrealistic goals?		Put things off until later?
	Fail to see the humor in situations others find funny?		Use sleeping pills and tranquilizers without a doctor's approval?
	Act rude?		Gossip?
	Make a "big deal" of everything?		Get angry when you are kept waiting?
	Look to other people to make things happen?		Think there is only one right way to do something?
	Have difficulty making decisions?		Complain you are disorganized?
	Fail to build relaxation time into your day?		Spend a lot of time complaining about the past?
	Avoid people whose ideas are different from your own?		Fail to get a break from noise and crowds?
	Keep everything inside?		Race through the day?
	Neglect exercise?		**TOTAL**

What does your score mean?

1–6: There are few hassles in your life, but don't avoid problems by shying away from challenges.

7–13: You are in fairly good control of your life. Work on the choices and habits that may be causing unnecessary stress in your life.

14–20: You are approaching the danger zone. You may be experiencing stress-related symptoms and strain in your relationships. Think carefully about choices you make and take time to relax every day.

Above 20: Emergency! You must take time now to work on your attitude, make changes to your diet, exercise, and relax.

("Stress Index" reproduced with permission from The Canadian Mental Health Association, Ottawa, Ontario, Canada)

Chapter Two
Stress And Your Health

Stress has numerous and far-reaching effects on both physical and mental health. The most obvious and commonly experienced symptoms of stress are headaches, insomnia, anxiety, stiff muscles, and upset stomach. Among the less-commonly known effects are impaired fertility, reduced sexual drive, and hampered immune function.

According to the American Psychological Association, 75 to 90 percent of all physician office visits are for stress-related ailments and complaints. Stress is linked to the six leading causes of death—heart disease, cancer, lung ailments, accidents, cirrhosis of the liver, and suicide. Following is a brief look at how stress impacts our health.

Aging

We have all seen people who go through stressful life events and seem to age before our eyes. Researchers have long thought that stress is a cause of premature aging, but the underlying mechanism was a mystery until recently when it was found that stress accelerates the aging process by damaging DNA.

Elizabeth Blackburn, PhD, and Elissa Epel, PhD, from the University of California, San Francisco, conducted a study to look at how real-life stress affects cellular aging.

Blackburn and Epel studied 39 women, ages 20 to 50, who had been experiencing intense stress because they were caring for a child suffering from a serious chronic illness, such as autism or cerebral palsy. They compared them to 19 women in the same age group whose children were healthy. Caregivers, especially those taking care of the ill, are typically in a high-stress category.

To look at the impact of stress on aging, the researchers examined a part of the DNA that controls cell aging, called a telomere. Blackburn discovered telomeres. She says, "If you think of a strand of DNA as a shoelace, the telomere is the plastic tip on the end. It protects the DNA from damage. Telomeres naturally get thinner as we age, and the thinner they get, the thinner the protection." When the telomeres fray away, the cell dies. That's why we lose eyesight, hearing, and muscle strength as we get older.

In their landmark study, Blackburn and Epel demonstrated that in women caring for a sick child, the telomeres shortened the equivalent of

10 years of premature aging compared to the control group. The longer a woman had been caring for a sick child, the shorter her telomeres, the lower her levels of telomerase (an enzyme that helps rebuild telomeres), and the higher her levels of "oxidative stress." Oxidative stress occurs when unstable molecules in the body called free radicals damage DNA, including telomeres. Telomerase levels naturally decline with age.

Also in this study, researchers found that the greater a woman's perception of her stress, the worse she scored on all these factors. The mothers who coped well under stress didn't suffer the same damage to their telomeres. This research points to the importance of having a healthy and positive attitude.

Cancer

Numerous studies have looked at the connection between stress and cancer, and some have reported that stress increases cancer risk. There may be several underlying factors at play here. Chronic stress weakens a person's immune system, which, in turn, may increase the risk of virus-associated cancers such as Kaposi sarcoma and some lymphomas.

Research in animals has found that the body's release of stress hormones into the blood in response to stimulation of the nervous system can directly alter important processes in cells that help protect against the formation of cancer, such as DNA repair and the regulation of cell growth. Studies have also indicated that stress can affect the growth and spread of tumors.

Cognitive Function

Cortisol, one of the adrenal hormones secreted during stress, while critical for our stress response, can have a variety of deleterious effects if secreted chronically and in excess. Cortisol excess can damage the nervous system, particularly the hippocampus, which is an area of the brain responsible for memory, concentration, and cognitive function. In extreme cases, it can compromise the ability of neurons (nerve cells) to survive oxidative stresses, resulting in neuron death. Stress is also one of the main underlying causes of insomnia, depression, and anxiety— all conditions that impair our cognitive function and emotional well-being.

Diabetes

Chronic stress has recently been implicated in the onset of diabetes. During periods of stress, the body enters a catabolic state in which it starts to break down tissue for energy. Additionally, blood glucose levels rise. This triggers the pancreas to release insulin, the hormone that brings glucose into our cells to be used for energy. However, the effects of insulin are

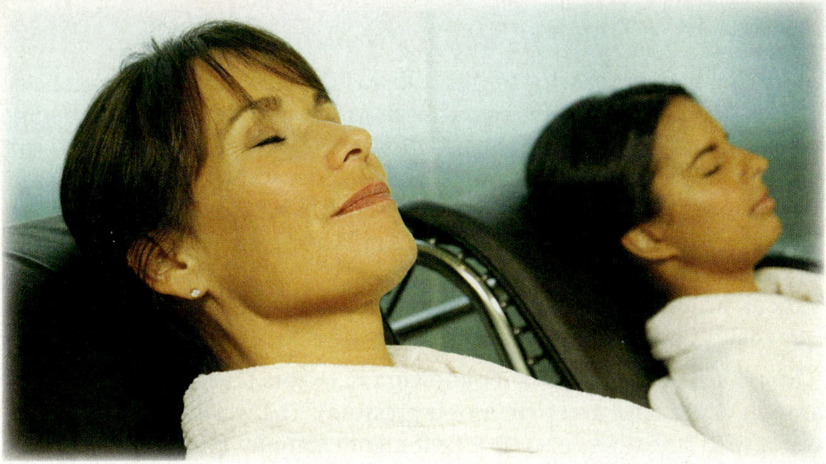

blunted by cortisol. The pancreas responds by pumping out more insulin, but as the body becomes less sensitive to its effects, insulin resistance occurs and blood glucose levels remain high. Insulin resistance and high blood glucose levels are the key features of type 2 diabetes, which is becoming a national epidemic. Those who are under stress and have other risk factors for diabetes, such as obesity, a sedentary lifestyle, and family history, should be screened twice a year by a health care practitioner.

Heart Disease

The connection between stress and heart disease has been recognized for many years. Heart attacks and sudden death happen more frequently following a tragedy or natural disaster. These events have both immediate and long-standing effects on heart health. In a study published in *Archives of General Psychiatry*, researchers found that Americans who said they became anxious and stressed after the 9/11 terrorist attacks (some just from watching the collapse of the twin towers on TV) reported higher rates of heart disease up to three years later. While several studies have found high rates of post-traumatic stress disorder and anxiety in first responders or attack survivors, most of the nearly 2,000 people randomly selected nationwide for this study had no direct connection to 9/11. The research showed that before September 11, 2001, about 22 percent of the participants reported they had heart ailments. Three years after the attacks, about 31 percent of them said they had developed heart problems. People who said they were stressed by the attacks were more than twice as likely to have high blood pressure one year after the attacks, and more than three times as likely to have heart problems two years after the attacks.

Heart disease is also much more common in individuals subjected to chronic stress, such as caring for a sick loved one. Researchers aren't sure exactly how stress increases the risk of heart disease. Stress itself might be an independent risk factor for heart disease because it exposes your body to unhealthy, persistently elevated levels of the stress hormones. The surge in adrenaline caused by severe emotional stress causes the blood to clot more readily, increasing the risk of heart attacks. British investigators have shown that chronic work stress can produce chronic increases in adrenaline levels, and have related those changes to an increased risk of heart disease. A Duke University study showed that the stress of performing difficult arithmetic problems can constrict the coronary arteries in such a way that blood flow to the heart muscle is reduced.

Stress can also worsen other known risk factors for heart disease (such as high cholesterol and high blood pressure). The way in which a person copes with stress may also be a factor. For example, some people smoke, overeat, or drink alcohol in excess when under stress, and these are all risk factors for heart disease.

Psychosocial factors, such as social isolation and even personality traits, may also be at play. Negative type A personality traits like anger, hostility, aggressiveness, time urgency, and inappropriate competitiveness are now recognized to be significant risk factors for heart attacks, elevated cholesterol and blood pressure, and stroke.

The Immune System

Have you noticed that you get sick during times of intense stress? That is because stress impairs the function of the immune system. Stress lowers your lymphocyte count and increases your body's production of free radicals. These effects weaken the immune system and increase the risk of infections. In fact, the most common causes of weakened immunity in healthy individuals are stress and aging. Studies have shown the higher the reported stress levels—whether measured by negative life change events, perceived stress level, or negative feelings—the higher the likelihood of developing a cold. A common finding is that the chance of physical illness increases with the number of life changes and the amount of stress experienced.

Sex

It is often said that sex is a great stress-reliever, and while there is truth to that, the problem is that stress in itself can dampen your sex drive or libido. In fact, stress has been identified as one of the leading causes of low libido for men and women. Stress causes a dramatic drop in testosterone levels, the key sex hormone that drives libido.

Stress is also a common cause of erectile dysfunction. In order for a man to have a healthy erection, there must be adequate blood flow to the penis. During stress, blood flow is directed to the arms and legs (not the genitals), making it difficult, if not impossible, for a man to get an erection.

Weight Gain

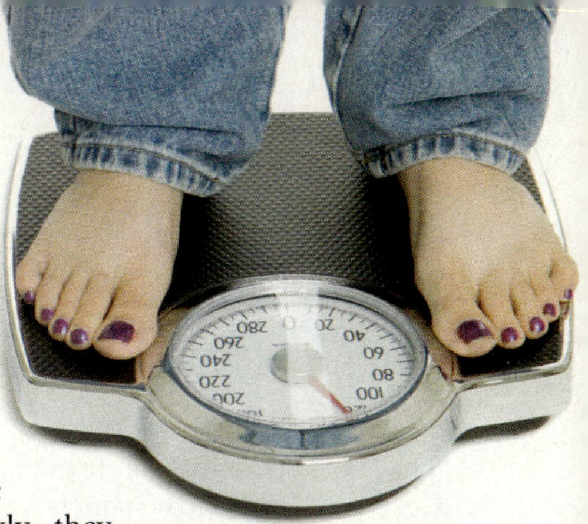

Weight gain, particularly around the midsection, is yet another consequence of chronic stress. Stress can trigger cravings for "comfort foods" such as high glycemic carbohydrates (breads, cookies, and other sweets). Not only are these foods high in calories (and excess calories mean weight gain), but since they break down into sugar quickly, they cause dramatic fluctuations in blood sugar levels. This triggers hunger, cravings for more sweets, and insulin spikes. As discussed earlier, perpetually high insulin levels can lead to insulin resistance (type 2 diabetes), but it can also impact your waistline. Insulin is a hormone that promotes fat storage—particularly around the midsection. Belly fat is now recognized to be closely tied to insulin resistance, and a risk factor for diabetes, heart disease, and certain cancers.

Like insulin, one of the functions of cortisol is to promote fat storage. During stress, cortisol helps to mobilize the body's energy stores. Cortisol can provide the body with protein for energy production through gluconeogenesis, the process of converting amino acids into useable energy (glucose) in the liver. It also can move fat from storage deposits and relocate it to fat cell deposits deep in the abdomen.

Another factor is that stress directly increases appetite. Again, one of the functions of cortisol is to help the body refuel in response to stress. However, in doing so, it keeps your appetite revved up, so you continually feel hungry. To make matters worse, researchers believe that cortisol directly influences food consumption by binding to receptors in the brain (specifically, the hypothalamus) that stimulate cravings for foods high in fat and/or sugar. Cortisol also indirectly influences appetite by regulating other chemicals that are released during stress, such as CRH (corticotrophin releasing hormone), leptin, and neuropeptide Y (NPY). High levels of NPY and CRH, and reduced levels of leptin, have been shown to stimulate appetite.

Lastly, levels of DHEA (dehydroepiandrosterone), testosterone, and growth hormone are reduced in response to stress. These hormones are involved in regulating muscle mass and metabolism, so when levels go down, it is bad news for your waistline as it leads to muscle loss and fat gain.

As you can see, stress has profound effects on health, influencing aging, risk for chronic disease, and body weight. In the next chapter, you will find some simple strategies that you can adopt to better manage stress.

Chapter Three

Stress Management Strategies

A successful program for managing stress is one that includes a holistic approach, namely stress management techniques, dietary modifications, exercise, sleep, and nutritional supplements. In this chapter, I will share with you my four-step plan for managing stress. You will learn how to identify your stressors; adopt strategies to take charge of your thoughts, attitude, and reactions; create balance; and find ways to accept the things you can't change so that you can enjoy a better quality life.

1. Identify Your Stressors

This first step in managing stress is to identify the sources of your stress, or your triggers. These are the thoughts or events that make you feel stressed, or the people who push your buttons. In order to do this, I would suggest keeping a journal or notepad handy so that when you feel stressed you can make a note of the circumstances. Whether it is situations at work or home, with family or friends, make a note of how you felt, how you reacted, and how you coped. Are your current coping strategies helpful, or do they make matters worse? Identifying your stressors and making notes of how you deal with stressful situations will help you in creating a stress management plan.

2. Adopt Stress Management Strategies

There are so many positive ways to deal with stress. Since we all have different triggers and different ways of responding to and coping with stress, you will need to experiment with the various techniques and strategies that I have outlined below. Keep in mind that you may need to adopt several of these strategies to help deal with your stressors. Adopt those that make you feel calm and in control. I would suggest trying one or two to start, and then gradually incorporating as many as you can into your life.

Avoid negative people and those who stress you out: the chronic complainers, those who never have anything nice to say, and those who seem to enjoy criticizing. If someone consistently makes you feel stressed to be around, limit the amount of time you spend with that person or end the relationship entirely.

Avoid the things that cause you the most stress, or find ways to alter stressful situations so that they are more tolerable. For example, if traffic is a trigger, see if you can change your work hours to minimize driving in rush hour or take a different route, even if it is longer. If that is not possible, try listening to music, news, or an audiobook while driving to make the time more enjoyable.

Train your mind to react differently to current triggers. Look at challenges in life as opportunities. This may take some time and practice. You will need to really examine how you think and react in various situations, and come up with ways to change your reactions. For example, if you find it stressful giving a speech, look at it as an opportunity to develop your public speaking skills. You can take a course or work with a coach, and with practice you will find speaking less stressful.

Develop a positive attitude. Positive thinking lessens stress, makes you feel happy, and makes others want to be around you. Start off by saying positive things to yourself each day: things you like about yourself, your achievements, your family, or your plans for the day. When feeling stressed, take time to reflect on all the positive things in your life.

Work on managing anger and hostility. This takes time. Practice controlling or redirecting your frustrations into something positive. If you have had a bad day at work, rather than get into a fight with your partner or children, go for a walk or a bike ride. This will help relieve the stress and put your energy into something more positive.

Take charge. Express your feelings and be assertive. This will make you feel more in charge and less like a victim of circumstances. Deal with problems up front; ignoring them or keeping them inside can lead to anger, resentment, feelings of helplessness, and anxiety. Work on communicating your thoughts and feelings with friends, family, or a counselor.

Look at the big picture. Sometimes we get caught up "stressing" over the small stuff. When faced with something causing you stress, ask yourself if it is really that important, whether it will matter in a week or month, and if it is worth getting upset over. If the answers are no, then let your worries and negative thoughts go and redirect your energy to things that matter.

Let go of perfectionism. Having high standards for yourself and others can set you up for unnecessary stress. Instead, set reasonable standards or expectations, and realize that perfection is not always achievable or necessary.

Learn to compromise. When in a dispute, finding some common ground or meeting a person halfway can leave both of you feeling more satisfied.

3. Create Balance

For many, working too much and not having time to relax and enjoy family and friends is a common source of stress, and can lead to burnout, frustration, anxiety, and sleeplessness. It is important to create balance in your life, take time for yourself, and engage in social activities. Here are some suggestions:

Schedule time for yourself each day, even if it is only a half hour. Set aside time to recharge your batteries and do something you enjoy, such as exercising, gardening, talking with friends, or taking a bath.

Learn to say no. Taking on more than you can handle and being overextended, either with work or other commitments, can lead to stress. Know your limits. Set boundaries and stick to them.

Work on improving your time management skills. Running late for appointments, squeezing too much into your day, and multitasking can be stressful. If your schedule is getting out of control, prioritize your activities and work on accomplishing only the most important items. Leave the extras for another day or cut them out completely. Delegating responsibilities is another helpful time management strategy. If you find large projects overwhelming, try breaking them down into smaller projects.

4. Accept The Things You Can't Change

Some sources of stress are unavoidable or beyond our control, such as dealing with a serious illness, losing a loved one, or living in hard economic times. These are events that you cannot change. In these cases, it is essential to gain acceptance of the situation and move forward. Dwelling on the negative leads to stress, frustration, and feelings of helplessness. Here are some points to keep in mind:

Rather than feeling stressed over things you cannot change, ***try to focus on the things that are in your control,*** such as your own thoughts, behaviors, and actions.

Look for the positives in a situation. Even during tough times, there are opportunities to learn and experience personal growth. Try reframing the problem and looking at it in a different light.

Learn to forgive. Holding a grudge or feeling angry and resentful leads to stress and negative emotions. While not always easy, work on forgiving and accepting.

Maintain a sense of humor. Being able to laugh at yourself when you make a mistake, and finding the humor and levity in challenging situations, is a great way to dissipate stress.

Chapter Four

Lifestyle Strategies

Now that you are aware of the value of stress management techniques and how to incorporate them into your life, let's take a look at the lifestyle strategies that effectively lessen stress: dietary approaches, exercise and relaxation techniques, and sleep.

Food And Mood

Your dietary choices have a significant impact on your emotional well-being and your ability to cope with stress. A healthy diet provides your body with sustained energy and the nutrients it needs to recuperate, regenerate, and repair. Conversely, an unhealthy diet can actually worsen your response to stress. So with that in mind, here are my top nutritional tips for combating stress:

Start your day right with breakfast. This really is the most important meal of the day. It will set the tone for how you feel, physically and emotionally. Try oatmeal with cinnamon and flaxseed, yogurt and berries, or poached eggs with whole-grain toast.

Eat small, frequent meals throughout the day. This will keep you energized and in a better position to deal with stress. In fact, it is much better to eat five small meals a day than three larger meals.

Choose low-glycemic carbohydrates such as whole-wheat pasta, whole-grain breads, brown rice, fruits, and vegetables. These foods provide essential nutrients needed to help the body deal with stress.

Ensure adequate protein intake. Protein provides sustained energy, and is required for muscle repair and growth. Choose lean poultry, fish, beans, legumes, nuts, and seeds.

Drink lots of purified water and calming herbal teas including chamomile, lemon balm, and passionflower.

Eat more fish, flaxseed, hemp, and chia seed. These foods contain essential fatty acids that are necessary for proper brain and nervous system function.

Foods to Avoid

High amounts of caffeine can trigger and worsen stress. Ironically, many people turn to coffee or soda when feeling stressed or tired. These beverages can actually increase the secretion of adrenaline and cortisol, making you more edgy and stressed. Plus, the temporary boost of energy is often followed by fatigue, leaving you in worse shape.

If you are currently drinking three or more cups of coffee daily, wean yourself from coffee slowly to avoid withdrawal symptoms. Caffeine withdrawal can be quite severe, causing irritability, depression, muscle pain, headaches, and anxiety. Try switching your morning coffee or soda to green tea. Green tea has much less caffeine, and contains an amino acid called L-theanine that promotes calming and relaxation. You can also get the benefits of L-theanine as a supplement under the brand name Suntheanine. This will be discussed in further detail in Chapter 5.

Many people turn to alcohol to relax, yet alcohol, like caffeine, can actually worsen the effects of stress. Alcohol is a diuretic, meaning it causes the body to lose water. The body senses dehydration as a stressor, and, as a result, cortisol levels rise. Alcohol can also impair sleep. Initially, an alcoholic drink may make you feel drowsy. However, it increases nighttime awakenings, thus impairing restorative sleep. Limit alcohol to one to two drinks per day.

Sugary foods cause fluctuations in blood sugar, which may cause mood swings and worsen the effects of stress. Cut down on candy, baked goods, snack foods, and products with added sugar and refined flour.

Fast food and processed foods (snack foods) are high in saturated fat and sugar, and low in nutritional value. These foods can trigger anxiety and mood swings.

Exercise For Less Stress

Regular physical activity plays a key role in reducing and preventing the effects of stress. In fact, the benefits of exercise in relieving stress are more powerful than any prescription drug. Clinical studies consistently show that exercise can ease tension and stress and cut the risk of almost every chronic disease.

When we exercise, there is a release of hormones called endorphins into the bloodstream. These hormones boost our mood, relieve stress, and improve our overall sense of well-being. Exercise improves blood flow to the brain, bringing additional sugars and oxygen that may be needed in times of mental strain. Increased blood flow to the muscles can help relax tense and sore muscles. Exercise also improves sleep quality, and getting a good night's sleep is critical for coping with stress.

Aside from the biochemical and physiological benefits of exercise, simply making the decision and effort to exercise can boost your self-image, distract you from stress and worry, and give you something positive and rewarding to focus on.

Studies have shown that physically fit people have less extreme physiological responses when under stress or pressure compared to those who are not fit. This means that exercise can act as a buffer against stress. Being fit can help you manage both the short- and long- term effects of stress, and minimize the adverse health effects of stress.

Make exercise a priority in your schedule and set aside one hour every day for exercise. If you don't have a one-hour block of time free, try to fit in two 30-minute activities. The benefits of exercise are cumulative, and every little bit helps. Going for a walk, stretching, riding a bike, dancing, or playing golf or tennis are just some of the ways to get the benefits of exercise. If you are currently not exercising, start slowly, and gradually increase the time and intensity. It is also recommended that you consult your health care practitioner before embarking on any new exercise program.

Yoga and tai chi are two forms of exercise that are particularly helpful for reducing stress.

Yoga

Yoga has been practiced for centuries by many cultures around the world. It is now recognized to be an effective method for reducing stress, improving flexibility and strength, and improving sleep and overall health.

The word yoga means "union" in Sanskrit, the language of ancient India where yoga originated. Yoga is the union occurring between the mind, body, and spirit. Yoga is about creating balance in the body through developing strength and flexibility. This is accomplished by performing poses or postures, each of which has specific physical benefits. The poses can be done quickly in succession, creating heat in the body through movement, or more slowly to increase stamina and perfect the posture of the pose. There are various types of yoga, and the approach varies depending on the tradition in which the teacher has been trained.

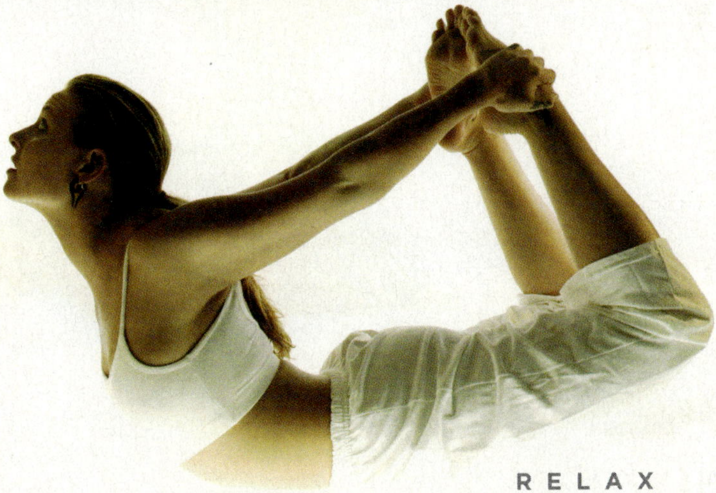

Yoga is a great activity for people of all ages. The best way to learn yoga is to join a class. There are many yoga DVDs that can be helpful, but in order to learn proper technique, seek the guidance of a qualified instructor. Once you learn the basics, yoga is something that you can practice on a mat in the comfort of your own home.

Tai Chi

Tai chi is a graceful form of exercise that was developed in China more than 2,000 years ago. Practiced regularly, tai chi can help reduce stress, increase flexibility, improve muscle strength and definition, increase energy, and improve feelings of well-being.

Tai chi is often described as "meditation in motion" because it promotes serenity through gentle movements, connecting the mind and body. It involves performing a series of postures or movements in a slow, graceful manner. Each posture flows into the next without pausing. Like yoga, tai chi is an activity that anyone, regardless of age or physical ability, can practice. To learn tai chi, it is best to seek the guidance of a qualified instructor. Group classes are affordable, and provide an opportunity to learn the techniques and enjoy social interaction.

Relaxation Techniques

In addition to a proper diet and regular exercise, consider the following relaxation techniques to take the edge off stress.

Massage

During stress, tension can build up in the muscles, causing a decrease in circulation and nutrient delivery to tissues that results in "knots" or sore muscles. These knots can be painful, inhibit your ability to perform daily tasks, and even impair sleep quality.

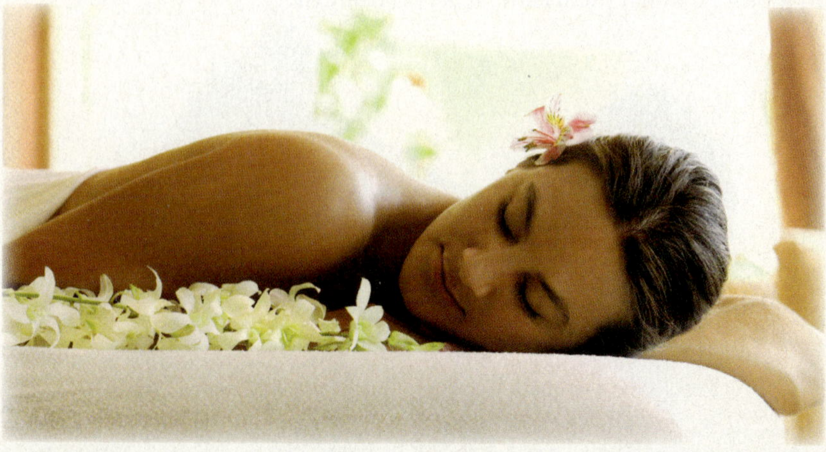

During a massage, a trained therapist rubs your body (often with oil) and manipulates your soft tissues (muscles, skin, and tendons). Massage increases blood flow to the muscles and tissues, which helps loosen stiff, sore muscles, promotes relaxation, increases the removal of metabolic waste, and promotes nutrient delivery to healing tissue. Massage can also boost your immune system, which may be compromised by chronic stress.

Massage can be performed by several types of health care professionals, such as a massage therapist, chiropractor, or physical therapist. Several versions of massage exist, such as Swedish massage, Shiatsu, aromatherapy massage, Thai massage, and sports massage. Many health plans cover massage therapy because of its recognized benefits for reducing stress and improving health.

Acupuncture

A treatment modality of traditional Chinese medicine, acupuncture is based on the philosophy that living beings have a vital energy, called "qi," that circulates through 12 invisible energy lines on the body known as meridians. Each meridian is associated with a different organ system. It is thought that an imbalance in the flow of qi throughout a meridian leads to disease and health problems.

According to Chinese medicine, stress, anxiety, depression, or any strong emotion interrupts the smooth flow of energy throughout the body. This can lead to pain, muscle tension, and other health problems. To restore balance to the flow of energy, an acupuncturist inserts needles into specified points along meridian lines. There are more than 1,000 acupuncture points on the body.

Western medicine has gradually come to accept and even endorse the benefits of acupuncture. Western practitioners believe that acupuncture works to alleviate stress by releasing endorphins (the natural pain-killing chemicals in the brain). Acupuncture also improves circulation of blood throughout the body, which oxygenates the tissues and cycles out cortisol and other waste chemicals. The calming nature of acupuncture also decreases heart rate, lowers blood pressure, and relaxes the muscles.

There are a variety of practitioners that offer acupuncture, such as traditional Chinese doctors, chiropractors, and physiotherapists. Like massage, many health plans now offer coverage for acupuncture.

Deep Breathing

During stress, many people hold their breath or take short shallow breaths from the chest rather than the abdomen. This can reduce oxygenation, lower energy levels, and worsen the effects of stress.

Deep breathing, also known as belly breathing or diaphragmatic breathing, is a simple yet effective stress reduction technique. This type of breathing increases oxygen levels in the body and has a natural calming effect.

This form of breathing can be done anytime and anywhere. To practice this technique, sit comfortably in a quiet area. Take a deep breath in through your nose, counting from one to four as you breathe in. Exhale through your mouth as you count down from four to one. Repeat 20 or 30 times. Try to practice deep breathing several times throughout the day, especially when you are feeling stressed.

Progressive Muscle Relaxation

Progressive muscle relaxation (PMR) is a relaxation technique that is helpful for relieving stress, muscle tension, insomnia, and even chronic pain. The technique involves tensing, or tightening one muscle group at a time, followed by a relaxation phase.

PMR can be practiced by nearly anyone at any age, and it requires only 10 to 20 minutes per day. Most practitioners recommend tensing and relaxing the muscle groups one at a time in a specific order, typically beginning with the lower extremities and working your way up to finish with the face. You can practice this technique seated or lying down. It is recommended that you practice PMR wearing comfortable clothing and in a quiet place free from distractions.

Begin by taking a deep breath in and contracting one muscle group (for example, your calves), for five to 10 seconds. Then, exhale and suddenly release the tension in that muscle group. Relax for 10 to 20 seconds, then move on to the next muscle group. Try to visualize your muscles relaxing and the stress flowing out of your body as you relax. With practice, you will find this technique very helpful for relieving stress and promoting calmness.

Visualization

Visualization, also known as mental imagery or guided imagery, is a method of connecting mind and body to promote relaxation and healing. It allows us to escape our stressful reality for a brief time and focus on thoughts that are calming and relaxing. To practice visualization, simply sit or lie down in a quiet, comfortable spot and close your eyes. Visualize a scene or place that makes you feel calm and happy. It could be a memory from childhood or a pleasurable vacation. Focus on the sights and sounds of this scene and imagine that you are there. Relax and enjoy.

Meditation

Meditation is a mental discipline that has been practiced for more than 5,000 years among Eastern cultures. It is a component of almost all religions. Today, it is commonly practiced in the West, outside of religion,

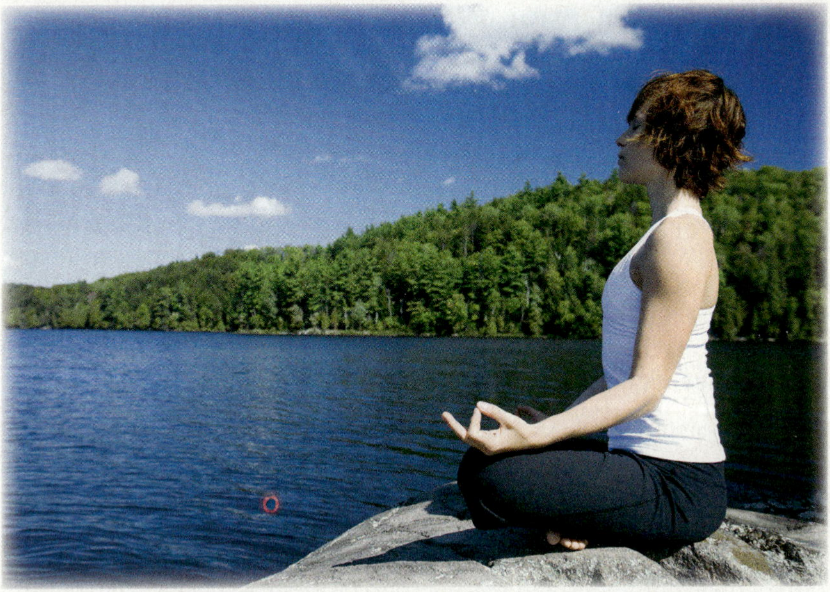

for stress management. Meditation involves turning attention to a single point of reference and entering into a deep state of relaxation. There are various meditative disciplines involving a wide range of spiritual and/or psychophysical practices. They emphasize different goals, including achieving a higher state of consciousness, greater focus, creativity, self-awareness, or simply a more relaxed and peaceful frame of mind.

Aside from promoting calmness, relaxation, and a sense of peace, meditation offers a number of other benefits: it slows heart rate and breathing, normalizes blood pressure, improves oxygenation, and reduces sweating. Meditation can lower cortisol levels, improve immune system function, and slow the aging process. It also helps clear the mind and boost creativity. Meditation has even been used to help people overcome addictions to alcohol, cigarettes, and drugs.

To meditate, go into a quiet area and sit in a comfortable chair, or cross-legged on the floor. Close your eyes and work on clearing your head. You may focus on a sound, like "om," or on your own breathing, or on nothing at all. Try to hush the inner voices and thoughts so that you can achieve internal silence. This is not easy to do, especially if you lead a busy lifestyle and are feeling stressed. It will take some practice, but eventually you will be able to let go of your thoughts and enjoy the feeling of relaxation. Allow 10 to 20 minutes to meditate.

Meditation is free, and it is something you can do anytime and anywhere. It takes some practice, but the time and effort are worthwhile.

Meditation is incredibly effective for reducing stress and improving emotional and physical well-being. The effects can be felt in just one session, but it also offers long-lasting benefits. If you need guidance, consult with an instructor.

Importance of Sleep

Sleep is one of our body's most basic and important needs. However, with our busy lifestyles, sleep deprivation is a common concern. In fact, nearly half of all adults report having difficulty sleeping. Stress and poor sleep go hand in hand: stress can affect our ability to get a good night's rest, and being tired and fatigued can impair our ability to cope with stress. When we are tired, we feel edgy, irritable, and are more reactive to stress.

Sleep is often thought of as a passive state, but it is during sleep that our body's major organs and regulatory systems are busy working on repair and regeneration. Hormones such as melatonin and growth hormone are secreted during sleep. Melatonin regulates our sleep cycles, and growth hormone is involved in tissue growth and repair. Sleep deprivation can impair production of these hormones, and this may be a factor in accelerated aging.

Sleep disorders are also more common with age, and our sleep patterns change with age (we spend less time in deep sleep). Researchers suspect that, in part, this may be the result of deteriorating sleep mechanisms associated with increased sensitivity to arousal-producing stress hormones, such as corticotropin-releasing hormone and cortisol. In one study, researchers compared patients with insomnia to those without sleep disturbances. They found that, "insomniacs with the highest degree of sleep disturbance secreted the highest amount of cortisol, particularly in the evening and nighttime hours." This suggests that chronic insomnia is a disorder of sustained hyperarousal of the body's stress response system.

Sleep deprivation has been linked to many serious diseases, including diabetes, heart disease, and cancer. According to Eve Van Cauter, PhD, a professor of medicine at the University of Chicago, "metabolic and endocrine changes resulting from a significant sleep debt mimic many of the hallmarks of aging. We suspect that chronic sleep loss may not only hasten the onset, but could also increase the severity, of age-related ailments such as diabetes, hypertension, obesity, and memory loss."

To improve your quality of sleep, work on developing good habits before bed that can affect sleep quality. Consider the following:

- Set aside at least seven to eight hours for sleep. Leaving only five or six hours for sleep may make you feel stressed and impact your ability to fall asleep.

- Establish a regular bedtime and wake time.
- Do relaxing activities before bed. For example, read a book, take a warm bath, or meditate.
- Reserve your bedroom for intimacy and sleep only; don't work in your bedroom.
- Make your bedroom dark, quiet, and comfortable.
- Exercise regularly, but not before bed. Exercise is stimulating, and when done too close to bedtime it can hamper sleep.
- Caffeine (coffee, tea, soda, and chocolate) can affect sleep quality, and should be avoided eight hours before bed.
- Alcohol may help you fall asleep, but it causes nighttime wakening and reduces sleep quality. Minimize alcohol consumption or avoid it completely.
- Go easy on sugary foods, especially in the evening. A "sugar-rush" can affect your ability to fall asleep.
- If you work the night shift or travel to different time zones, try supplementing with melatonin (a hormone naturally secreted in response to darkness that helps promote sleep).

Supplements containing L-theanine (specifically Suntheanine) can improve sleep quality and also reduce stress. "Suntheanine is the only substance, natural or otherwise, that reduces feelings of stress and improves sleep quality without creating drowsiness or diminished motor performance," explains Michael R. Lyon, MD, Medical and Research Director of the Canadian Center for Functional Medicine with the University of British Columbia. "Because of this, I am currently studying the benefits of Suntheanine in 100 boys with attention deficit hyperactivity disorder (ADHD)."

Unhealthy Coping

When faced with stress, avoid self-medicating with alcohol, cigarettes, or drugs. These substances may seem to provide an easy escape from stress, but the relief is only temporary, and chronic and excessive use of these substances is damaging. Alcohol stimulates the secretion of the stress hormone adrenaline, resulting in problems such as nervousness, irritability, and insomnia. Alcohol can weaken the immune system and impair the ability of the liver to remove toxins from the body. Smoking damages the nervous system, worsens stress, and hampers sleep quality. It is also linked to many other chronic diseases such as cancer, heart disease, and lung disease.

Chapter Five

Stress-Busting Supplements

As mentioned in the beginning of this booklet, a solid program for managing stress is one that includes a holistic approach, utilizing stress management techniques, dietary approaches, relaxation methods, exercise, and supplements. This chapter highlights the role of supplements. The proper supplements can offer significant benefits by helping to control and lessen the effects of stress, reduce cortisol levels, improve mental function and clarity, and improve sleep.

Foundation Products

There are three key supplements that I recommend as the foundation for your stress management program.

Multivitamin-mineral complex

In order to function properly, our bodies require an adequate supply of vitamins, minerals, and trace elements. While we can obtain some of these nutrients from food, there are many reasons why it is important to take a daily "multi":

- Our food supply provides lower levels of nutrients today due to changes in soil quality and growing conditions.
- Our nutritional habits have drastically changed over the past few decades; people eat more fast-food, convenience foods, and packaged foods which have less nutritional value compared to whole, fresh, unprocessed foods.
- Stress depletes vitamins and minerals in the body, particularly the B-vitamins, vitamin C, calcium, and magnesium.
- Pollution, toxins, and certain prescription drugs deplete nutrients in the body.
- A multi helps ensure that your body gets all the essential nutrients it needs to function optimally.

Our nutrient needs vary with age, gender, health status, and lifestyle factors such as our activity level and whether we smoke. Multivitamins come in a wide range of formulas. Look for a product that provides 50 to 100 mg of the B vitamins. The B vitamins have been known for decades as the "stress vitamins" because of the vital role they play in the health of the nervous system and in adrenal function. They act as coenzymes in numerous metabolic reactions in the body. Niacin (vitamin B3) is required for tryptophan metabolism, and tryptophan is a precursor to serotonin (a neurotransmitter that calms the mind). Vitamins B6 and B12 are necessary for the integrity of the nerves. Pantothenic acid (vitamin B5) plays an important role in stress relief. B vitamins can be depleted by stress, and a deficiency can actually cause anxiety and worsen the response to stress. For assistance in choosing the right multi for you, talk to a pharmacist or health care practitioner.

Omega-3 fatty acids

Omega-3 fatty acids are required for the health and function of the brain and nervous system. These essential fatty acids are incorporated into the cell membranes. They influence how cells communicate and support neurotransmitter function. Omega-3 fatty acids are found in fish and seeds (chia, flax, and hemp seeds). Fish is the preferred source because it contains higher amounts of the biologically active fatty acids, eicosapentaenoic acid (EPA) and docosahexaenoic acid (DHA). Omega-3 fatty acids may help with the management of stress, and they also reduce your risk of developing coronary heart disease, one of the more severe conditions that you can develop from too much stress. Dosage: 3 to 6 grams daily.

L-theanine

Over the past few decades, countless studies have revealed that the antioxidants in green tea benefit heart health, cancer prevention, weight loss, digestion, cognitive function, immune function, and more. But there is another component of green tea that is gaining popularity—the amino acid L-theanine. L-theanine occurs naturally in tea plants, and is found in the highest concentration in green tea leaves. It creates the characteristic "umami" flavor, also known as the "fifth taste" (besides the four traditional tastes: sweet, salty, acid, and bitter).

L-theanine offers a wide range of benefits for stress management: it promotes calming and relaxation, improves sleep quality, and heightens mental clarity and focus. And it offers all of this without causing any serious side effects, drowsiness, tolerance, or addiction. While it may sound too good to be true, numerous studies have validated the benefits of L-theanine, and it is now regarded as one of the safest and most effective natural products for stress.

"The form of L-theanine is very important," explains researcher Michael Lyon, MD. "I strongly advise my patients to look for products that contain Suntheanine." Lyon, with the University of British Columbia, says "Any other products are probably impure and cannot be trusted. I know that Suntheanine is produced in Japan to meet the highest standards of purity and it is the only L-theanine that has been studied in dozens of published clinical trials."

There are a few ways in which L-theanine helps to alleviate stress and improve mental function. It is absorbed from the intestine, enters the bloodstream, and crosses into the brain. There, it exerts subtle changes in biochemistry: it increases production of GABA, a neurotransmitter that blocks the release of dopamine and serotonin, resulting in reduced stress and anxiety. Second, L-theanine directly stimulates production of alpha waves in the brain, creating a state comparable to meditation in which there is deep relaxation yet mental alertness. Third, research suggests that L-theanine has neuroprotective effects in the brain, particularly in preventing neuronal (nerve cell) death in the hippocampus, a key area impacted by the effects of stress. Lastly L-theanine is a caffeine antagonist, offsetting the stimulant (anxiety-provoking) properties of caffeine without causing drowsiness.

Suntheanine is a patented, pure form of L-theanine developed by Taiyo International Inc. that has been specifically studied for its health benefits. More than 100 clinical studies have been conducted on this branded ingredient. Here is a summary of some of the key benefits that have been identified in studies of Suntheanine:

- **Stress:** reduces symptoms of stress and anxiety; promotes calmness
- **Cognitive function:** improves mental focus, clarity, alertness, reaction time, and memory
- **Sleep:** improves sleep quality; reduces nighttime awakenings and nightmares
- **PMS:** reduces irritability, anger, and mood swings
- **ADHD:** improves sleep quality, reduces hyperactive behaviors, and improves short-term memory
- **Immune System:** improves immune function; reduces incidence of cold/flu
- **Heart health:** lowers blood pressure

The recommended dosage of Suntheanine is 50 to 200 mg. The effects of Suntheanine are generally felt within 30 minutes, and have been shown to last eight to 12 hours. Suntheanine is not impacted by food; it can be taken at any time. There are several high-quality dietary supplements available that feature Suntheanine as a key ingredient.

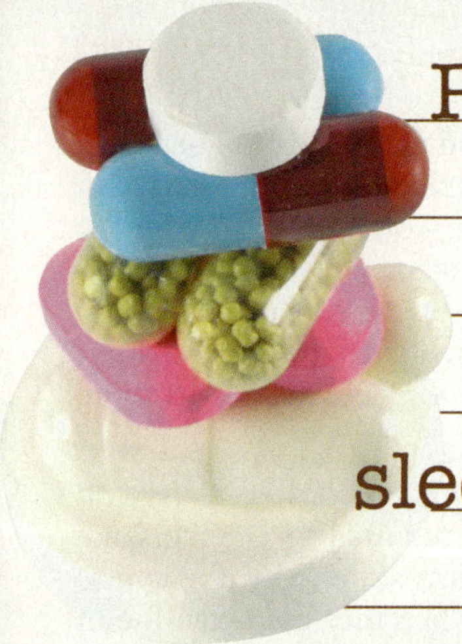

Prescription drugs can impair sleep quality, and we know that poor sleep makes us more reactive to stress.

Supportive Products

Following is a list of some other supplements to consider for managing stress and/or sleep. It is not necessary to take all of these products. They each work differently and offer various benefits. Review your options and talk to your health care practitioner for guidance in choosing the right products.

Panax Ginseng: an adaptogenic herb that helps reduce the response to stress. It also supports physical and mental performance, immune function, and adrenal gland function, all of which can be hampered by stress. Dosage: 100 to 200 mg daily.

Vitamin C: helps the adrenal glands in dealing with the stress response. Vitamin C is involved in the production of neurotransmitters that are required for mood and proper sleep. It also provides support for the heart and immune system (areas impacted negatively by stress). Vitamin C levels are depleted by stress, smoking, and use of birth control pills. Dosage: 500 to 1,000 mg daily.

Valerian: an herb that has sedative properties. It is helpful for managing occasional insomnia, but it may cause next-day drowsiness. The dosage varies depending on the formulation (tablet or tincture), so check with a health care practitioner before taking this product.

Melatonin: a hormone naturally secreted from the pineal gland in the brain that regulates our sleep-wake cycles. Supplements of synthetic melatonin have been studied and found to be helpful for improving sleep quality in those working night shifts or traveling to different time zones. Dosage: 3 to 6 mg one hour before bed.

Prescription Drugs

The main class of drugs used to treat stress and anxiety are the benzodiazepines, namely alprazolam (Xanax), clonazepam (Rivotril), diazepam (Valium), and lorazepam (Ativan). These drugs work quickly (within 30 to 60 minutes) to ease anxiety and promote relaxation. However, they have numerous side effects, including drowsiness, loss of coordination, dizziness, and memory impairment. To make matters worse, these drugs can impair sleep quality, and we know that poor sleep makes us more reactive to stress.

Benzodiazepines are highly addictive, and some people can develop a tolerance (which means a higher dosage is required to get the same effect). Unfortunately, I have seen many patients suffer with the consequences of relying on prescription sedatives. When they are taken for an extended period of time (more than two weeks) they become habit-forming. Discontinuation can cause horrible withdrawal symptoms, such as heightened anxiety, confusion, memory loss, and even seizures—making matters worse than before the drug was taken.

Drugs that are often prescribed for stress, especially when it occurs with depression and/or anxiety, are the selective serotonin reuptake inhibitors (SSRIs), which include fluoxetine (Prozac), sertraline (Zoloft), fluvoxamine (Luvox), paroxetine (Paxil), and citalopram (Celexa). More prescriptions are dispensed for antidepressants—232.7 million nationwide in 2007—than for drugs of any other type, according to the data firm IMS Health. In 2007, sales of antidepressants totaled $11.9 billion in the United States.

Since women are more likely to see their doctors when feeling stressed, anxious, or depressed, and also more likely to talk about their feelings, it is not surprising that they are the most medicated. In fact, twice as many psychotropic drugs (drugs that affect the mind) are prescribed for women as for men. According to a report issued by the Center for Mental Health Services of the Centers for Disease Control and Prevention, more than one in three doctor's office visits by women involved a prescription for an antidepressant.

While antidepressant drugs help some people, their benefits are often exaggerated and their side effects and risks minimized. Case in point: a 2008 report published in the *New England Journal of Medicine* revealed that many drug companies selectively publish only studies showing positive benefits with their drugs, skewing the overall results and misleading doctors and patients. It was found that in published trials, about 60 percent of people taking prescription drugs report significant relief from depression, compared with roughly 40 percent of those on placebo pills. But when the less positive, unpublished trials are included, the advantage shrinks: the drugs outperform placebos, but by a modest margin. Another review of antidepressant drug studies conducted by psychologist Irving Kirsch, PhD, came to the same conclusion: "The overall difference between medication and placebo was so small that it was clinically insignificant for all but the most depressed patients."

Side effects of the SSRIs include nausea, weight gain/loss, headaches, anxiety, nervousness, insomnia or drowsiness, diarrhea, sweating, tremor, and sexual dysfunction. These drugs also have numerous potential drug interactions, so if you are taking them it is important to consult with a pharmacist before taking any other prescription or natural product.

Please note: You should never discontinue a prescription drug without first consulting with your doctor.

In Conclusion

Stress is an unavoidable part of life. It's critical to find healthy ways to relax because if we don't manage stress properly, it can take a serious toll on our health. Through a combination of diet, lifestyle, and dietary supplements, we can avoid dangerous prescription drugs and ward off the negative health effects of chronic stress.

Selected References

American Psychological Association: "Stress in America," News release, *American Psychological Association*, Oct. 24, 2007.

Ashton H. Psychotropic drug prescribing for women. *British Journal of Psychiatry* 158 (suppl.10):30-35,1997.

Bukowski J. L-theanine intervention enhances human gamma delta T lymphocyte function. *Nutr Rev* 66(2):96-102, Feb 2008.

Cavagnini F, et al. Glucocorticoids and neuroendocrine function. *International Journal of Obesity* 24: S77-S79, 2000.

Epel ES, et al. Accelerated telomere shortening in response to life stress. *Proc Natl Acad Sci USA* 101(49):17312-5, Dec 1, 2004.

Epel ES, et al. Stress and body shape: stress-induced cortisol secretion is consistently greater among women with central fat. *Psychosomatic Medicine* 62:623-632, 2000.

Epel E, et al. Stress may add bite to appetite in women: a laboratory study of stress-induced cortisol and eating behavior.*Psychoneuroendocrinology* 26:37-49, 2001.

Haskell CF. The effects of L-theanine, caffeine and their combination on cognition and mood. *Biol Psychol* 77(2):113-22, Feb 2008.

Holman EA, et al. Terrorism, Acute Stress, and Cardiovascular Health. A 3-Year National Study Following the September 11th Attacks. *Arch Gen Psychiatr* 65(1):73-80, 2008.

Kirsch I, et al. Initial Severity and Antidepressant Benefits: A Meta-Analysis of Data Submitted to the Food and Drug Administration. *PLoS Med* 5(2), 2008.

National Cancer Institute, Psychological Stress and Cancer. http://www.cancer.gov/cancertopics/factsheet/Risk/stress

Rogers PJ. Time for tea: mood, blood pressure and cognitive performance effects of caffeine and theanine administered alone and together. *Psychopharmacology* 195(4):569-577, Jan 2008.

Rowe CA, et al. Specific Formulation of Camellia sinensis Prevents Cold and Flu Symptoms and Enhances T Cell Function: A Randomized, Double-Blind, Placebo-Controlled Study. *Journal of the American College of Nutrition* 26(5):445–452, 2007.

Spiegel K, et al., Impact of sleep debt on metabolic and endocrine function. *The Lancet* 354:1435-1439, 1999.

Timmcke J. Efficacy (against premenstrual syndrome) and short term safety of L-theanine in a randomized, double-blind, parallel-group study in humans. Data on file, Taiyo International Inc.

Tomlinson JW, and Stewart PM. The functional consequences of 11 Beta- hydroxysteroid dehydrogenase expression in adipose tissue. *Hormone and Metabolism Research* (11-12) 34:746-751, 2002.

Turner EH, et al. Selective Publication of Antidepressant Trials. *N Engl J Med* 358:2180-2182, 2008.

Vgontzas AN, et al. Chronic Insomnia Is Associated with Nyctohemeral Activation of the Hypothalamic-Pituitary-Adrenal Axis: Clinical Implications. *Journal of Clinical Endocrinology and Metabolism* 86(8):3787-3794, April 2001.

For more information about the products mentioned, visit:

www.suntheanine.com

For more information about the author of this booklet, visit:

www.sherrytorkos.com

better nutrition *magazine presents*

RELAX

POWERFUL **STRESS REDUCTION** STRATEGIES

Stress is an unavoidable part of life, but if we don't properly manage it, it can take a serious toll on our health. That's why it's critical to develop positive coping measures including diet and lifestyle approaches and scientifically-studied dietary supplements. In this booklet, holistic pharmacist Sherry Torkos shows readers how to successfully cope with life's many stressors. Torkos provides a wide variety of proven stress-reducing strategies that will help readers relax and enjoy life. Torkos also gives advice on safe and natural alternatives to prescription tranquilizers and sedatives. Even though we can count on having stress in our lives, the comprehensive relaxation approach Torkos describes will help mitigate its effects and keep our body and mind healthy.

ABOUT THE AUTHOR OF THIS BOOKLET

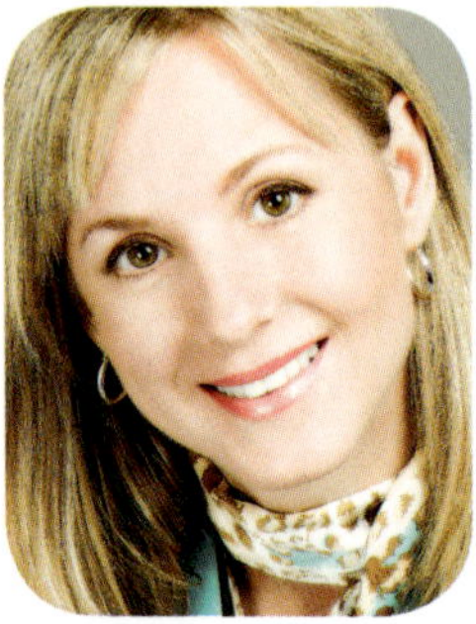

Sherry Torkos is a practicing pharmacist, author, and certified fitness instructor. She received her bachelor of science in pharmacy from the Philadelphia College of Pharmacy and Science. Sherry is actively involved in providing education on natural health matters and is frequently interviewed on radio and TV talk shows throughout North America and abroad. Sherry has authored 11 books, including *The Canadian Encyclopedia for Natural Medicine*, *The GI Made Simple*, and *Winning at Weight Loss*.

ISBN: 978-1-935297-14-7

50495

9 781935 297147

better nutrition healthy living guide

betternutrition.com